The Lasting Journey to a Healthier You

Sustainable Weight Loss Strategies after forty (40)

By

Justin C. Wilson

Disclaimer

Acknowledgments

Writing a book is never a solitary endeavor, and the completion of "The Lasting Journey to a Healthier You" is no exception. I am profoundly grateful to the many individuals and sources of inspiration that made this book possible.

First and foremost, I would like to express my gratitude to my family for their unwavering support throughout this journey. Your encouragement and understanding during the late nights and weekends spent writing were invaluable.

I extend my heartfelt appreciation to the experts in the fields of nutrition, fitness, and psychology who generously shared their knowledge and insights. Your expertise has enriched the content of this book and will undoubtedly benefit countless readers.

To the individuals who shared their personal weight loss stories and experiences, you are the real heroes of this book. Your candidness and determination serve as powerful examples of what can be achieved through dedication and resilience.

A special thanks to my editor and the publishing team who meticulously polished this manuscript and helped shape it into its final form. Your guidance and expertise were indispensable.

I also want to acknowledge the countless authors, researchers, and health professionals whose work has informed and influenced the content of this book. Your contributions to the field of health and wellness are immeasurable.

To my readers, thank you for embarking on this journey with me. Your quest for a healthier and happier life is a testament to your strength and determination.

Lastly, I want to express my deepest appreciation to all those who believe in the power of knowledge and the pursuit of better health. May this book serve as a valuable resource on your path to lasting well-being.

With gratitude,

Justin C. Wilson

Table of content

Introduction

In the grand tapestry of life, the age of 40 often marks a significant crossroads. It's a juncture where wisdom and experience converge, where we reflect on our accomplishments and perhaps, reassess our priorities. For many, it's also a time when health and wellness take center stage. As we navigate the ever-evolving landscape of our bodies, one of the most common aspirations is achieving a sustainable weight loss journey that can carry us into our golden years with vitality and vigor.

"The Lasting Journey to a Healthier You: Sustainable Weight Loss Strategies after 40" is a guidebook crafted to illuminate the path toward healthier living and sustainable weight loss for those who have reached this pivotal stage in life. It's a book for those who are ready to embark on a transformative journey, embracing the challenges and triumphs of achieving and maintaining a healthy weight, not just for the present, but for the rest of their lives.

In the pages that follow, we will explore the unique challenges that individuals face when striving for weight loss after the age of 40. We will delve into the physiological changes that occur with age and how they impact our metabolism, energy levels, and overall well-being. Understanding these changes is the first step in crafting a tailored and effective strategy for sustainable weight loss.

However, this book is not just about the science of aging and weight loss; it's about empowering individuals to take charge of their health and happiness. It's about instilling the belief that it's never too late to transform your life, to shed excess weight, and to embrace a healthier, more vibrant version of yourself.

"The Lasting Journey to a Healthier You" takes a holistic approach to weight loss, addressing not only the physical aspects but also the emotional and psychological factors that play a pivotal role in our relationship with food and our bodies. We will explore mindfulness techniques, stress management, and strategies for overcoming the emotional hurdles that often accompany the quest for weight loss.

Furthermore, this book will guide you through sustainable lifestyle changes, emphasizing the importance of balanced nutrition, regular physical activity, and long-term habit formation. These are the pillars upon which lasting health and wellness are built.

Throughout this journey, you will encounter inspiring success stories, practical tips, and expert advice from renowned nutritionists, fitness trainers, and individuals who have triumphed over the challenges of weight loss after 40. Their stories will serve as beacons of hope and motivation, reminding you that your goals are not only achievable but also well within your reach.

"The Lasting Journey to a Healthier You" is not a quick-fix solution but rather a roadmap to a healthier and more fulfilling life. It's a testament to the resilience of the human spirit and the boundless potential that resides within each of us. It's an invitation to embark on a journey of self-discovery, transformation, and empowerment.

So, dear reader, as you turn the page to embark on this voyage toward a healthier you, remember that you are not alone. Within these words, you will find the guidance and support you need to navigate the challenges of weight loss after 40, and with determination and commitment, you will discover a brighter, healthier future awaiting you on the other side. Welcome to "The Lasting Journey to a Healthier You."

Chapter 1

Embracing Your Health Transformation After 40

The Significance of Age 40

The age of 40 is a significant milestone in many people's lives, often marked by a unique combination of personal reflection and physical change. While it may not have the same cultural significance as turning 18 or 21, it holds a distinctive place because it represents a critical juncture in the journey of adulthood. Here's a closer look at the significance of age 40:

Self-Reflection: At 40, individuals tend to engage in deep self-reflection. They take stock of their life's achievements, goals, and the path they've traveled. It's a moment for introspection, where one may assess their career, relationships, and personal aspirations.

Midlife Transition: Age 40 often coincides with what is commonly referred to as a "midlife crisis" or, more positively, a "midlife transition." This is a time when people reevaluate their life choices, make adjustments, and seek new experiences or challenges.

Health Awareness: As people enter their 40s, health becomes a primary concern. They become more conscious of their physical well-being and may undergo routine medical check-ups, and screenings, and adopt healthier lifestyles. It's a pivotal age for health awareness.

Physical Changes: The 40s are marked by noticeable physical changes. Metabolism tends to slow down, making weight management more challenging. Individuals may experience changes in their vision, muscle mass, and energy levels, which can impact their daily lives.

Parenting and Empty Nest Syndrome: Many people in their 40s are parenting or are experiencing the "empty nest" phase as their children leave home for college or start their own lives. This shift in family dynamics can bring both relief and emotional adjustments.

Career Reevaluation: Age 40 often prompts a reevaluation of one's career. Some may seek career changes, while others may explore entrepreneurship or pursue passions they had set aside earlier in life.

Financial Planning: People in their 40s typically focus more on financial planning and saving for retirement. The realization that retirement is not too far off encourages financial prudence.

Embracing Wisdom: With four decades of life experience, individuals in their 40s often feel a sense of wisdom and maturity. They may find that they approach challenges and decisions with a greater sense of perspective and calm.

Personal Growth: The 40s can be a time of personal growth and self-discovery. People may pursue new hobbies, take up learning endeavors, or engage in personal development to continue evolving as individuals.

Reconnecting with Passions: Many individuals use this phase to reconnect with passions and interests that may have been neglected during the demands of earlier adulthood, bringing a sense of fulfillment and joy.

Age 40 represents a pivotal moment in life where individuals engage in introspection, make important decisions, and prioritize health and well-being. It's a time of transformation and self-discovery, and how one navigates this period can have a profound impact on the years to come.

Setting Realistic Goals for Sustainable Health

Setting realistic goals for sustainable health is a crucial step in any journey toward well-being, especially as we reach the age of 40 and beyond. Realistic goals provide a clear roadmap for progress, motivate us to stay on track and increase the likelihood of long-term success. Here's a guide on how to set realistic health goals:

Assess Your Current Health: Start by evaluating your current health status. Consider factors like your weight, fitness level, diet, sleep quality, stress levels, and any existing health conditions. This baseline assessment will help you identify areas that need improvement.

Be Specific: Your goals should be specific and well-defined. Rather than a vague goal like "I want to be healthier," specify what you want to achieve. For example, "I want to lose 20 pounds," "I want to run a 5k race," or "I want to reduce my daily sugar intake to under 30 grams."

Set Measurable Objectives: Your goals should be measurable so that you can track your progress. Use concrete metrics like pounds lost, inches reduced, minutes of exercise per day, or servings of vegetables eaten. Measurable goals allow you to celebrate milestones along the way.

Attainability: Ensure your goals are attainable within a reasonable timeframe. Consider your current lifestyle, commitments, and any physical limitations. Setting overly ambitious goals can lead to frustration and burnout. Gradual, sustainable changes are often more effective.

Relevance: Your goals should align with your overall health and well-being. Ask yourself why each goal matters to you. Understanding the significance of your goals can motivate you during challenging times.

Time-Boun: Set a timeframe for achieving your goals. Having a deadline creates a sense of urgency and helps you stay focused. However, make sure the timeframe is realistic. Rapid, extreme changes are seldom sustainable.

Break Down Larger Goals: If your ultimate goal is significant, break it down into smaller, more manageable steps. This makes the journey less daunting and allows you to celebrate achievements more frequently.

Consider Accountability: Share your goals with a trusted friend, family member, or a health professional. Having someone to hold you accountable can be a powerful motivator.

Adaptability: Life is unpredictable, and setbacks are inevitable. Be prepared to adjust your goals as needed. Flexibility is key to maintaining motivation and preventing discouragement.

Track Your Progress: Keep a journal or use a tracking app to monitor your progress. Regularly review your achievements and make any necessary adjustments to your plan.

Reward Yourself: Celebrate your successes, no matter how small. Rewards can help reinforce positive behaviors and make the journey more enjoyable.

Seek Professional Guidance: If you have complex health goals or underlying medical conditions, consult with healthcare professionals, such as a doctor, nutritionist, or personal trainer, to create a tailored plan.

Remember that the path to sustainable health is a marathon, not a sprint. By setting realistic, achievable goals and embracing gradual, positive changes, you'll be better equipped to maintain a healthy lifestyle well into your 40s and beyond.

The Mindset for Lasting Change

Achieving lasting change, especially when it comes to health and well-being after the age of 40, is as much about mindset as it is about physical action. Developing the right mindset can be the foundation for sustainable transformation. Here are key principles for cultivating the mindset for lasting change:

Self-Reflection: Start by understanding your current mindset and beliefs about change. Are you open to it, or do you resist it? Self-reflection allows you to identify any mental barriers that may be hindering your progress.

Embrace Positivity: Maintain a positive outlook. Instead of focusing on what you're giving up, concentrate on the benefits of the change. Visualize your success and the positive impact it will have on your life.

Set Realistic Expectations: Recognize that change takes time and effort. Be patient with yourself and avoid expecting instant results. Unrealistic expectations can lead to frustration and disappointment.

Accept Imperfection: Understand that setbacks are a natural part of the change process. Don't view them as failures but as opportunities to learn and adjust your approach. Perfection is not required for progress.

Develop Resilience: Cultivate resilience to bounce back from setbacks and challenges. Resilience involves adaptability and the ability to persevere in the face of difficulties.

Focus on Process, Not Perfection: Concentrate on the daily actions and habits that lead to change, rather than fixating on the result. A process-oriented approach encourages consistency and long-term success.

Practice Self-Compassio: Be kind and compassionate to yourself. Avoid self-criticism and negative self-talk. Treat yourself as you would treat a friend facing a similar challenge.

Mindfulness and Awareness: Practice mindfulness to stay present and aware of your thoughts, feelings, and behaviors. Mindfulness can help you make conscious choices aligned with your goals.

Seek Support: Don't hesitate to seek support from friends, family, or support groups. Sharing your journey with others can provide encouragement, accountability, and a sense of community.

Learn from Failure: Failure is not a dead-end but a stepping stone to success. Analyze what went wrong, adjust your strategy, and continue moving forward with newfound knowledge.

Celebrate Small Wins: Acknowledge and celebrate every small achievement along the way. These milestones provide motivation and reinforce the belief that change is possible.

Develop a Growth Mindset: Embrace the concept of a growth mindset, where you believe that your abilities and intelligence can be developed through dedication and hard work. This mindset encourages resilience and a willingness to learn.

Stay Committed: Commitment to your goals is crucial for lasting change. Remind yourself regularly of your "why" – the reasons behind your desire for change.

Visualize Success: Use visualization techniques to imagine yourself successfully achieving your goals. This mental rehearsal can enhance your confidence and motivation.

Keep Learning: Continue to educate yourself about the changes you're making. Knowledge empowers you to make informed decisions and adapt to new challenges.

Changing your mindset is a journey in itself. It may take time to shift your perspective and develop the mental resilience needed for lasting change. Be patient with yourself, stay persistent, and believe in your ability to transform your health and well-being in your 40s and beyond. Your mindset can be your greatest asset on this journey.

Chapter 2

Understanding the Science of Aging and Weight Loss

How Your Metabolism Changes with Age

Metabolism, the complex process by which your body converts food and drink into energy, does indeed change with age. As you reach your 40s and beyond, several factors contribute to a slowdown in metabolism. Here's an overview of how metabolism changes with age:

Basal Metabolic Rate (BMR) Decline: BMR represents the number of calories your body needs to maintain basic functions like breathing and cell repair at rest. It tends to decrease with age, primarily because muscle mass tends to decrease as well. Muscle tissue burns more calories at rest than fat tissue, so less muscle means a slower metabolism.

Hormonal Changes: Hormonal shifts play a significant role. With age, there's a decline in hormones like estrogen and testosterone, which can affect metabolism. These hormonal changes can lead to a redistribution of fat, often accumulating around the abdomen.

Reduced Physical Activity: As people age, they tend to become less active. A sedentary lifestyle can lead to muscle loss and a decrease in physical activity-related calorie expenditure. This further contributes to a slower metabolism.

Digestive System Changes: Aging can lead to changes in the digestive system, such as decreased stomach acid production, which can affect nutrient absorption. This may impact the efficiency of calorie utilization.

Loss of Lean Body Mass: Beyond just muscle loss, there can be a decrease in overall lean body mass, including bone density. This can further reduce calorie-burning capacity.

Dietary Choices: As people age, dietary habits may change. Some may consume fewer calories due to a decreased appetite, while others may opt for less nutrient-dense foods, which can impact metabolism.

Insulin Resistance: Insulin resistance tends to increase with age, making it harder for cells to take up glucose from the bloodstream. This can lead to higher blood sugar levels and potential weight gain.

Thermic Effect of Food (TEF) Reduction: TEF refers to the calories your body spends digesting and metabolizing the food you eat. It can decrease with age, meaning that your body may become less efficient at burning calories through digestion.

Changes in Circadian Rhythms: Disruptions in sleep patterns and circadian rhythms, which can become more common with age, may also affect metabolism and the regulation of hunger and satiety hormones.

Note that while metabolism generally slows with age, the degree of change varies from person to person. Genetics, lifestyle factors, and overall health play significant roles in how your metabolism evolves.

To counteract the natural slowdown in metabolism that comes with age, it's crucial to adopt a healthy lifestyle that includes regular physical activity, strength training to preserve muscle mass, a balanced diet, and adequate sleep. These habits can help mitigate the effects of age-related metabolic changes and promote overall well-being. Consulting with a healthcare professional or nutritionist can also provide personalized guidance to support a healthy metabolism as you age.

Hormonal Shifts and Their Impact

Hormonal shifts are a natural part of the aging process, and they can have a significant impact on various aspects of your health and well-being, especially as you reach your 40s and beyond. These hormonal changes are driven by factors like genetics, lifestyle, and, in the case of women, menopause. Here's an overview of hormonal shifts and their impact:

Menopause in Women:

- Estrogen Decline: Menopause, typically occurring in the late 40s or early 50s, marks the end of a woman's reproductive years. During menopause, there's a significant decline in estrogen production. This hormonal change can lead to various physical and emotional symptoms, including hot flashes, night sweats, mood swings, and changes in bone density.

- Weight Distribution: Changes in hormonal balance can affect the distribution of body fat. Many women experience weight gain, particularly around the abdomen, during and after menopause.

- Metabolic Impact: The decrease in estrogen can contribute to a decrease in metabolic rate, making it more challenging to maintain or lose weight.

- Bone Health: Estrogen plays a crucial role in maintaining bone density. Its decline can lead to a higher risk of osteoporosis and fractures. Bone health has become a significant concern for postmenopausal women.

Testosterone in Men and Women:
- Testosterone Decline: Both men and women experience a gradual decline in testosterone levels with age. While testosterone is often associated with men, it's also present in women and plays a role in various aspects of health.
- Muscle Mass and Strength: Lower testosterone levels can contribute to the loss of muscle mass and strength, affecting physical performance and metabolic rate.
- Mood and Energy: Testosterone can influence mood and energy levels. A decrease in testosterone may lead to fatigue, reduced motivation, and mood changes.
- Sexual Health: In both sexes, testosterone is linked to sexual health. Reduced levels can result in decreased libido and sexual function.

Thyroid Hormones:

- Thyroid Function: Thyroid hormones, which regulate metabolism, can also change with age. Some individuals may develop hypothyroidism (underactive thyroid) or other thyroid disorders, which can impact energy levels, weight, and overall well-being.

Insulin and Glucose Regulation:
- Insulin Sensitivity: Aging can lead to reduced insulin sensitivity, potentially resulting in higher blood sugar levels and an increased risk of type 2 diabetes.

While these hormonal shifts are a natural part of aging, their effects can be influenced by factors like genetics, lifestyle choices, and overall health. Additionally, not everyone will experience the same degree of hormonal changes or the same symptoms.

To mitigate the impact of hormonal shifts on your health and well-being, consider the following:
- Maintain a healthy lifestyle with regular exercise and a balanced diet.
- Seek medical guidance for managing specific hormonal issues or conditions.
- Pay attention to your mental and emotional well-being and seek support when needed.

- Prioritize bone health through weight-bearing exercises and adequate calcium and vitamin D intake.
- Be proactive in managing any chronic health conditions or risk factors.

Consulting with a healthcare provider, such as an endocrinologist or gynecologist, can provide personalized guidance on managing hormonal changes and their impact on your overall health as you age.

Muscle Mass and Its Role in Weight Management

Muscle mass plays a pivotal role in weight management, especially as we age. Understanding the significance of muscle in maintaining a healthy weight and metabolism is essential, particularly for those over the age of 40. Here's how muscle mass influences weight management:

Metabolism and Calorie Burning: Muscle tissue is metabolically active, meaning it burns calories even at rest. This is referred to as your Basal Metabolic Rate (BMR). Having more lean muscle mass increases your BMR, allowing you to burn more calories throughout the day, even when you're not actively exercising. As you age, preserving and building muscle becomes crucial for maintaining a healthy metabolism.

Weight Loss and Fat Loss: When you're trying to lose weight, the goal is typically to reduce body fat while preserving lean muscle mass. If you lose weight through calorie restriction or crash diets without incorporating strength training exercises, you may lose muscle along with fat. This can lead to a less favorable body composition and a slower metabolism.

Physical Function and Mobility: Maintaining muscle mass is essential for overall physical function and mobility. As we age, the loss of muscle mass and strength can lead to decreased mobility, balance issues, and an increased risk of falls and injuries.

Insulin Sensitivity: Muscle tissue plays a key role in glucose metabolism. Having more muscle can improve insulin sensitivity, which helps regulate blood sugar levels. Improved insulin sensitivity can reduce the risk of type 2 diabetes and facilitate weight management.

Bone Health: Strength training exercises that build muscle also stimulate bone growth and maintenance.

This is particularly important for older adults, as it can help prevent or mitigate osteoporosis and reduce the risk of fractures.

Appetite Regulation: Muscle tissue produces various hormones and peptides that play a role in appetite regulation. Having adequate muscle mass may help regulate hunger and prevent overeating.

To enhance the role of muscle mass in weight management, consider the following strategies, especially if you're over 40:

- Incorporate Strength Training: Engage in regular strength training exercises, such as weight lifting or bodyweight exercises, to build and maintain muscle mass. Aim for at least two to three sessions per week.

- Balanced Nutrition: Consume a balanced diet that provides adequate protein to support muscle maintenance and repair. Protein-rich foods like lean meats, poultry, fish, dairy, and plant-based sources like beans and tofu are essential.

- Adequate Caloric Intake: Avoid extreme calorie restriction, which can lead to muscle loss. Instead, focus on creating a modest calorie deficit through a combination of diet and exercise for sustainable weight loss.

- Hydration: Stay adequately hydrated to support muscle function and recovery.
- Rest and Recovery: Ensure you get sufficient rest and sleep, as this is when your body repairs and builds muscle tissue.
- Consult a Professional: If you have specific weight management goals or concerns related to muscle loss, consider consulting a registered dietitian, personal trainer, or healthcare provider for personalized guidance.

Building and maintaining muscle mass is a gradual process. Consistency in strength training and a holistic approach to nutrition and lifestyle are key to achieving and maintaining a healthy body composition and effective weight management, especially as you age.

Chapter 3

Navigating Emotional Challenges and Eating Habits

Emotional Eating and Coping Strategies

Emotional eating is a common behavior where individuals use food to cope with their emotions, such as stress, sadness, boredom, or anxiety. While it's natural to seek comfort in food from time to time, chronic emotional eating can lead to weight gain and negative emotional cycles. Developing healthier coping strategies is essential, especially for those over the age of 40 who may be more susceptible to stressors. Here are some strategies to manage emotional eating:

Recognize Triggers: The first step in addressing emotional eating is to identify your triggers. Keep a journal to track when and why you turn to food for emotional comfort. Recognizing patterns can help you become more aware of your behaviors.

Mindful Eating: Practice mindful eating by paying attention to what you eat, when you eat, and why you eat. Pause before reaching for food and ask yourself if you're genuinely hungry or if there's an emotional trigger at play.

Find Alternative Coping Mechanisms: Instead of turning to food, explore alternative ways to cope with emotions. Engage in activities you enjoy, such as reading, walking, listening to music, or practicing relaxation techniques like deep breathing or meditation.

Emotion Regulation: Work on improving your emotional regulation skills. This may involve seeking therapy or counseling to learn how to manage and process emotions more healthily.

Social Support: Reach out to friends, family, or support groups when you're feeling overwhelmed emotionally. Sharing your feelings with others can provide comfort and reduce the need for emotional eating.

Healthy Snacking: If you find yourself reaching for snacks when you're not truly hungry, opt for healthier options like fruits, vegetables, or a small portion of nuts. This can satisfy cravings without excessive calorie intake.

Meal Planning: Plan regular, balanced meals and snacks throughout the day to prevent extreme hunger, which can trigger emotional eating. Ensure your meals contain a mix of protein, fiber, and healthy fats to keep you satisfied.

Remove Temptations: Keep unhealthy, tempting foods out of your immediate environment. Stock your pantry and fridge with nutritious options, making it easier to make healthy choices when emotional eating strikes.

Stress Management: Find effective ways to manage stress, such as exercise, yoga, or journaling. Reducing stress can significantly reduce the urge to eat for emotional comfort.

Professional Help: If emotional eating is causing significant distress and interfering with your quality of life, consider seeking help from a therapist, counselor, or registered dietitian who specializes in emotional eating.

Practice Self-Compassion: Be kind to yourself and avoid self-criticism. Understand that emotional eating is a common behavior, and setbacks can happen. Treat yourself with the same compassion you would offer a friend.

Set Realistic Goals: Focus on making gradual changes in your eating habits and emotional coping strategies. Set realistic goals to address emotional eating over time rather than trying to eliminate it.

Addressing emotional eating is a process that may require patience and practice. It's essential to be gentle with yourself as you work towards healthier ways of managing your emotions. Developing a toolbox of coping strategies can significantly reduce the reliance on food for emotional comfort and promote a more balanced and emotionally healthy lifestyle.

Mindful Eating: Connecting with Your Food*****

Mindful eating is a practice that encourages you to fully engage with your food, savor each bite, and develop a deeper connection with the act of eating. This practice goes beyond simply consuming calories; it involves being present and attentive during meals. Here's how to cultivate mindful eating habits and connect more meaningfully with your food:

Create a Calm Environment: Choose a quiet, calm setting for your meals, free from distractions like TV, smartphones, or work. Create a pleasant atmosphere that encourages you to focus on your food.

Engage Your Senses: Pay attention to the sensory aspects of your meal. Notice the colors, textures, and aromas of the food on your plate. Take a moment to appreciate the visual and olfactory aspects of your meal.

Eat Slowly: Slow down the pace of your eating. Put your utensils down between bites, chew slowly, and savor the flavors. Eating more slowly allows you to better enjoy each bite and recognize when you're satisfied.

Chew Thoroughly: Take the time to thoroughly chew your food. This not only aids in digestion but also allows you to fully experience the taste and texture of what you're eating.

Savor Each Bite: Be mindful of the taste sensations in your mouth. Notice the subtle flavors, the interplay of sweet, salty, sour, and bitter tastes. Try to identify different ingredients and spices.

Listen to Your Body: Tune into your body's hunger and fullness cues. Before eating, ask yourself if you're truly hungry. During the meal, periodically check in with your body to determine if you're satisfied or if you need more.

Eat with Gratitude: Take a moment to express gratitude for the food in front of you. Acknowledge the effort that went into preparing the meal and the nourishment it provides.

Mindful Portion Control: Be aware of portion sizes and serve yourself a reasonable amount. Mindful eating can help prevent overeating by allowing you to recognize when you've had enough.

Pause and Reflect: Midway through your meal, pause for a moment. Reflect on how you feel physically and emotionally. Are you still hungry, or are you satisfied? This pause allows you to make conscious choices about whether to continue eating.

Practice Non-Judgment: Be kind to yourself and avoid judgment or criticism about your food choices. Mindful eating is about fostering a non-judgmental awareness of your eating habits.

Observe Emotions: Pay attention to the emotional aspects of eating. Are you eating out of habit, stress, or boredom? Mindful eating encourages you to recognize emotional triggers and choose healthier ways to cope.

Stay Hydrated: Drink water throughout your meal to stay hydrated and help with digestion. Be mindful of your thirst signals as well as your hunger signals.

Appreciate the Journey: Consider the journey of your food, from its source to your plate. Think about the people, processes, and resources that contributed to your meal.

Mindful eating can foster a more positive relationship with food, promote healthier eating habits, and even aid in weight management. By connecting with your food more deeply and mindfully, you can derive greater enjoyment from your meals and develop a healthier approach to nourishing your body.

Overcoming Common Psychological Barriers

Overcoming common psychological barriers is essential for making lasting changes in various aspects of life, including health, relationships, and personal growth. These barriers can hinder progress and hold you back from reaching your goals, especially as you age. Here are some common psychological barriers and strategies to overcome them:

Fear of Failure: The fear of failing can paralyze you and prevent you from even trying. To overcome this barrier:

- Reframe failure as a learning opportunity.

- Set realistic goals and celebrate small successes along the way.

- Cultivate a growth mindset, where you see challenges as opportunities for growth.

Self-Doubt: Negative self-talk and self-doubt can erode your confidence. To combat self-doubt:

- Challenge negative thoughts with evidence of your abilities and past successes.

- Surround yourself with supportive and positive people.

- Seek professional help if self-doubt is persistent and debilitating.

Procrastination: Procrastination can keep you from taking action on your goals. To overcome it:

- Break tasks into smaller, manageable steps.

- Set deadlines and hold yourself accountable.

- Use time-management techniques like the Pomodoro method.

Perfectionism: Striving for perfection can lead to paralysis and dissatisfaction. To tackle perfectionism:

- Embrace a "good enough" mindset. Aim for progress, not perfection.

- Recognize that mistakes are part of the learning process.

- Prioritize self-compassion over self-criticism.

Lack of Motivation: A lack of motivation can be a significant barrier to change. To boost motivation:
  - Identify your "why" – the underlying reasons for your goals.
  - Break goals into smaller, more manageable tasks to maintain momentum.
  - Find inspiration in role models or success stories.

Negative Self-Image: A negative self-image can hinder your confidence and self-esteem. To improve self-image:
  - Practice self-acceptance and self-compassion.
  - Challenge unrealistic beauty standards and societal pressures.
  - Seek professional help if a negative self-image is deeply ingrained.

Cognitive Biases: Cognitive biases, such as confirmation bias or all-or-nothing thinking, can distort your perception and decision-making. To counter cognitive biases:
  - Be aware of common cognitive biases and actively challenge them.
  - Seek diverse perspectives and information to counter confirmation bias.

- Practice open-mindedness and flexibility in your thinking.

Overcoming Comfort Zones: Fear of stepping out of your comfort zone can limit personal growth. To expand your comfort zone:
- Gradually expose yourself to new experiences and challenges.
- Focus on the potential rewards and personal growth that come from pushing boundaries.
- Develop a growth mindset that embraces change and adaptability.

Social Pressure: The expectations and judgments of others can be a significant psychological barrier. To navigate social pressure:
- Clarify your values and priorities to guide your decisions.
- Set boundaries and communicate your needs assertively.
- Surround yourself with supportive and like-minded individuals.

Lack of Patience: Impatience can lead to frustration and discouragement. To foster patience:
- Set realistic timelines for your goals.

- Remind yourself that change takes time and effort.
- Celebrate small milestones along the way to maintain motivation.

Overcoming psychological barriers requires self-awareness, persistence, and often a willingness to seek support from friends, family, or professionals. Remember that it's normal to face these barriers, but with the right strategies, you can break through them and achieve your goals, even as you age.

Chapter 4

Building a Balanced Nutrition Foundation

Nutritional Needs After 40

As you age, your nutritional needs may change, and it becomes increasingly important to make informed dietary choices to support your health and well-being. Here are some key nutritional considerations and needs to focus on after the age of 40:

Caloric Intake: Metabolism tends to slow down with age, which means you may require fewer calories than you did in your younger years. Adjust your calorie intake based on your activity level, and be mindful not to overconsume calories, which can lead to weight gain.

Protein: Protein is essential for maintaining and building muscle mass, especially as muscle loss can occur with age. Include lean protein sources such as poultry, fish, beans, legumes, and low-fat dairy products in your diet.

Calcium and Vitamin D: Both calcium and vitamin D are crucial for maintaining bone health, which becomes increasingly important as you age. Dairy products, fortified foods, leafy greens, and supplements, if necessary, can help ensure you get enough of these nutrients.

Fiber: Fiber is essential for digestive health and can help manage weight and lower the risk of chronic diseases. Increase your fiber intake by consuming whole grains, fruits, vegetables, and legumes.

Omega-3 Fatty Acids: Omega-3 fatty acids are known for their anti-inflammatory properties and can support heart and brain health. Fatty fish like salmon, walnuts, flaxseeds, and chia seeds are good sources of omega-3s.

Antioxidants: Antioxidants, such as vitamins C and E, can help combat oxidative stress and support healthy aging. Incorporate a variety of colorful fruits and vegetables into your diet to ensure you get a range of antioxidants.

Hydration: Staying hydrated is important for overall health, especially as you age. Dehydration can lead to a range of health issues, so be sure to drink enough water throughout the day.

Iron: Iron needs to decrease for postmenopausal women, but men should still be mindful of their iron intake. Lean meats, poultry, fish, and fortified cereals can provide adequate iron.

B Vitamins: B vitamins are important for energy metabolism and brain function. Whole grains, leafy greens, nuts, and lean meats are good sources of B vitamins.

Potassium: Potassium is essential for heart and muscle health. Foods like bananas, potatoes, oranges, and leafy greens are rich in potassium.

Folate: Folate is necessary for cell division and repair. Leafy greens, legumes, and fortified foods are good sources of folate.

Limit Added Sugars and Processed Foods: As you age, it's even more important to limit added sugars and highly processed foods. These can contribute to weight gain and chronic health conditions.

Portion Control: Pay attention to portion sizes to avoid overeating and maintain a healthy weight. As metabolism slows, it's easier to gain weight if you're not mindful of portion control.

Consult with a Healthcare Professional: Individual nutritional needs can vary widely based on factors like genetics and health conditions. It's advisable to consult with a registered dietitian or healthcare professional to create a personalized nutrition plan that addresses your specific needs and goals.

Maintaining a balanced diet, staying physically active, and making healthy lifestyle choices are key components of supporting your overall health and well-being as you age. Nutrition plays a crucial role in promoting vitality, preventing chronic diseases, and maintaining a high quality of life in your 40s and beyond.

Crafting a Sustainable Meal Plan

Creating a sustainable meal plan is a key step in maintaining a healthy and balanced diet, especially as you age. Here's a step-by-step guide to crafting a meal plan that is not only nutritious but also sustainable and enjoyable:

Set Clear Goals: Begin by defining your nutritional and health goals. Consider factors like weight management, managing chronic conditions, improving energy levels, and overall well-being. Having clear goals will guide your meal planning.

Assess Your Current Diet: Take a look at your current eating habits. Identify areas where you might need to make improvements. Are you getting enough fruits and vegetables? Are you consuming too much processed or high-sugar foods? Understanding your starting point is essential.

Diversify Your Diet: Aim for variety in your meal plan to ensure you get a wide range of nutrients. Include a colorful array of fruits and vegetables, whole grains, lean proteins, and healthy fats. Diversification also keeps your meals interesting and enjoyable.

Balanced Macronutrients: Ensure your meal plan includes a balance of macronutrients – carbohydrates, proteins, and fats. This balance provides sustained energy and supports overall health.

Portion Control: Pay attention to portion sizes to avoid overeating. Use measuring cups, plates, or the "hand method" (e.g., a palm-sized portion of protein) to help estimate appropriate portions.

Regular Eating Schedule: Stick to a regular eating schedule with balanced meals and snacks spaced throughout the day. This can help regulate blood sugar levels and prevent overeating later in the day.

Plan Ahead: Plan your meals and snacks for the week. Create a shopping list based on your plan to avoid impulse purchases of unhealthy foods. Preparing meals in advance can also save time and reduce reliance on less healthy convenience foods.

Include Healthy Snacks: Incorporate nutritious snacks like Greek yogurt with berries, a handful of nuts, or cut-up veggies with hummus between meals to maintain energy levels and curb overeating during main meals.

Hydration: Don't forget about staying hydrated. Aim to drink plenty of water throughout the day. Sometimes, thirst can be mistaken for hunger.

Mindful Eating: Practice mindful eating by paying full attention to your meals. Avoid eating in front of the TV or computer and savor each bite. This can help you recognize when you're satisfied and prevent overeating.

Flexibility: Allow for flexibility in your meal plan. It's okay to enjoy occasional treats or dine out without guilt. A sustainable meal plan accommodates occasional indulgences.

Listen to Your Body: Pay attention to hunger and fullness cues. Eat when you're hungry and stop when you're satisfied. Avoid eating out of habit or emotional triggers.

Seek Professional Guidance: If you have specific dietary concerns or health conditions, consult with a registered dietitian or healthcare professional. They can provide personalized guidance and ensure your meal plan meets your unique needs.

Evaluate and Adjust: Periodically assess how your meal plan is working for you. Are you meeting your goals? Do you feel energized and satisfied? Adjust your plan as needed based on your evolving needs and feedback from your body.

A sustainable meal plan is one that you can maintain over the long term. It should not be overly restrictive or cause unnecessary stress. Focus on making gradual, positive changes to your eating habits that support your health and well-being well into your 40s and beyond.

The Role of Macronutrients and Micronutrients

Macronutrients and micronutrients are essential components of a balanced diet, each playing a unique role in maintaining overall health and well-being, especially as you age.

Macronutrients:

Carbohydrates:

- Role: Carbohydrates are the body's primary source of energy. They provide fuel for daily activities and bodily functions.

- Types: Carbohydrates can be categorized as simple (sugars) and complex (starches and fiber). Complex carbohydrates are more slowly digested and provide sustained energy.

- Sources: Whole grains, fruits, vegetables, legumes, and dairy products are excellent sources of carbohydrates.

Proteins:

- Role: Proteins are essential for building and repairing tissues, producing enzymes and hormones, and supporting the immune system. They are also a source of energy when needed.

- Sources: Lean meats, poultry, fish, dairy products, eggs, beans, nuts, and tofu are rich in protein.

Fats:

- Role: Dietary fats are necessary for energy storage, absorption of fat-soluble vitamins (A, D, E, and K), and overall cellular function. Omega-3 and omega-6 fatty acids, found in certain fats, are important for heart and brain health.

- Types: Fats can be categorized as saturated, unsaturated (monounsaturated and polyunsaturated), and trans fats. Unsaturated fats, especially from sources like avocados, nuts, and fatty fish, are considered heart-healthy.

- Sources: Healthy fat sources include avocados, nuts, seeds, olive oil, and fatty fish like salmon and mackerel.

Micronutrients:

Vitamins:

- Role: Vitamins are essential for various biochemical processes in the body. They support immunity, vision, bone health, and skin health, among other functions.

- Examples: Vitamin A (found in carrots and sweet potatoes), vitamin C (found in citrus fruits), vitamin D (synthesized in the skin with sunlight exposure), and vitamin K (important for blood clotting) are examples of vitamins.

Minerals:

- Role: Minerals are essential for maintaining healthy bones, muscles, and overall bodily functions. They play roles in nerve function, fluid balance, and oxygen transport.

- Examples: Calcium (crucial for bone health and found in dairy products), iron (essential for transporting oxygen in the blood), potassium (important for heart and muscle function), and magnesium (involved in over 300 enzymatic reactions) are examples of minerals.

Trace Elements:

- Role: Trace elements are minerals required in very small amounts but are still crucial for health. They include selenium, zinc, copper, and iodine, among others.

- Sources: Trace elements are typically obtained through a balanced diet and are found in foods like seafood, nuts, and whole grains.

Antioxidants:

- Role: Antioxidants, such as vitamin C, vitamin E, and beta-carotene, help protect cells from oxidative damage caused by free radicals. They play a role in reducing the risk of chronic diseases and supporting immune function.

- Sources: Fruits, vegetables, nuts, and seeds are rich sources of antioxidants.

Balancing macronutrients and micronutrients in your diet is essential for maintaining overall health and preventing nutritional deficiencies. A varied and balanced diet that includes a wide range of food groups will help ensure you get the necessary macronutrients and micronutrients to support your well-being, especially as you age. Consulting with a registered dietitian or healthcare provider can provide personalized guidance based on your specific nutritional needs and goals

Chapter 5

Exercise and Fitness for Lasting Health

Age-Appropriate Exercise Routines

Maintaining an age-appropriate exercise routine is crucial for promoting physical fitness, flexibility, and overall well-being as you age. Here are some exercise recommendations tailored to different age groups:

In Your 40s:

Cardiovascular Exercise: Engage in at least 150 minutes of moderate-intensity aerobic exercise or 75 minutes of vigorous-intensity exercise per week. Activities like brisk walking, jogging, swimming, or cycling can help improve heart health and maintain a healthy weight.

Strength Training: Include strength training exercises at least two days a week. This can involve lifting weights, using resistance bands, or bodyweight exercises. Strength training helps preserve muscle mass and metabolism.

Flexibility and Mobility: Incorporate regular stretching and mobility exercises to maintain flexibility. Yoga and Pilates are excellent options for improving flexibility and balance.

Core Work: Focus on core exercises to support posture and stability. Planks, bridges, and abdominal exercises can help strengthen your core muscles.

In Your 50s:

Cardiovascular Exercise: Continue cardiovascular exercise, but consider low-impact options like swimming or stationary cycling to reduce joint stress. Aim for the same weekly duration as in your 40s.

Strength Training: Maintain or increase strength training to counteract age-related muscle loss. Focus on full-body workouts that target major muscle groups.

Balance and Stability: Incorporate balance and stability exercises into your routine. These can include single-leg exercises, balance boards, or Tai Chi. Improving balance reduces the risk of falls.

Joint Health: Pay attention to joint health. Warm up properly before exercising, and consider adding joint-friendly supplements like glucosamine and chondroitin if recommended by a healthcare professional.

In Your 60s and Beyond:
Cardiovascular Exercise: Continue with cardiovascular activities, but be mindful of any limitations or joint issues. Listen to your body and choose exercises that are comfortable and safe.

Strength Training: Focus on maintaining muscle mass and bone density. Lighter weights or resistance bands may be appropriate. Include balance and flexibility exercises to prevent injuries.

Low-Impact Activities: Consider low-impact activities such as water aerobics, gentle yoga, or Tai Chi, which are easier on the joints and still provide cardiovascular benefits.

Functional Training: Emphasize functional training exercises that mimic everyday movements, such as squats, lunges, and stepping exercises. This helps maintain the ability to perform daily tasks independently.

Consult a Healthcare Professional: If you have any medical conditions or concerns, consult with a healthcare provider or physical therapist for personalized exercise recommendations and modifications.

Regardless of your age, it's essential to prioritize safety during exercise. Warm up before workouts, listen to your body, and stop any activity that causes pain or discomfort. Always consult with a healthcare provider before starting a new exercise program, especially if you have any underlying health conditions or concerns.

Remember that consistency is key to reaping the benefits of exercise as you age. Regular physical activity can enhance your quality of life, maintain independence, and contribute to your overall health and well-being throughout your life.

Strength Training and Cardiovascular Health

Strength training and cardiovascular exercise each offer unique benefits for your health, and when combined, they create a well-rounded fitness routine that can have a profound impact on your overall well-being, including cardiovascular health. Here's how strength training and cardiovascular exercise contribute to heart health:

Strength Training:
Muscle Mass: Strength training helps build and maintain muscle mass. As your muscle mass increases, your body becomes more efficient at burning calories, which can aid in weight management and reduce the risk of obesity, a major risk factor for heart disease.

Metabolism: An increase in muscle mass can boost your resting metabolic rate. This means you burn more calories even when you're not exercising, supporting weight control and overall metabolic health.

Blood Pressure: Some studies have shown that regular strength training can lead to reductions in resting blood pressure, which is a key indicator of cardiovascular health. Lower blood pressure reduces the strain on your heart.

Blood Sugar Regulation: Strength training can improve insulin sensitivity, helping your body better regulate blood sugar levels. This is particularly important for reducing the risk of type 2 diabetes, which is closely linked to heart disease.

Cholesterol Levels: While cardiovascular exercise is more directly associated with improving cholesterol profiles, strength training can still have a positive impact. It may help increase levels of HDL (the "good" cholesterol) and reduce levels of LDL (the "bad" cholesterol).

Cardiovascular Exercise:

Heart Health: Cardiovascular exercise, also known as aerobic exercise, directly targets the heart and circulatory system. It strengthens the heart muscle, improves its efficiency, and enhances overall cardiovascular function.

Blood Pressure: Regular aerobic exercise can lower both resting and exercise-induced blood pressure. It helps keep blood vessels flexible and reduces the risk of hypertension.

Cholesterol: Cardiovascular exercise can significantly improve cholesterol profiles by increasing HDL cholesterol and decreasing LDL cholesterol and triglycerides. This contributes to a healthier cardiovascular system.

Weight Management: Aerobic exercise is an effective way to burn calories and manage body weight, which is crucial for heart health.

Maintaining a healthy weight reduces the risk of heart disease.

Reducing Inflammation: Chronic inflammation is a risk factor for heart disease. Cardiovascular exercise can help reduce inflammation markers in the body.

To maximize cardiovascular benefits and overall health, consider incorporating both strength training and cardiovascular exercise into your fitness routine. The American Heart Association recommends at least 150 minutes of moderate-intensity aerobic exercise or 75 minutes of vigorous-intensity aerobic exercise per week, along with muscle-strengthening activities on two or more days per week.

A balanced exercise routine that includes strength training and cardiovascular exercise can enhance heart health, improve metabolic function, and reduce the risk of cardiovascular diseases. Remember to consult with a healthcare provider or fitness professional before starting a new exercise program, especially if you have any underlying medical conditions or concerns.

Incorporating Physical Activity into Daily Life

Incorporating physical activity into your daily life is a great way to stay active and improve your overall health, especially if you have a busy schedule or find it challenging to commit to regular workouts. Here are some practical tips for integrating more physical activity into your daily routine:

Take Short Walks: Whenever you have a break or some free time during the day, take a short walk. It could be a walk around your office building, a stroll in your neighborhood, or even a few laps around your home.

Use Active Transportation: Whenever possible, choose active transportation methods like walking or cycling instead of driving for short trips or commuting to work. This not only adds physical activity to your day but also reduces your carbon footprint.

Take the Stairs: Opt for stairs instead of elevators or escalators whenever you can. Climbing stairs is an excellent way to strengthen your legs and boost your heart rate.

Break Up Sedentary Time: If you have a desk job, make it a habit to stand up and stretch or walk around for a few minutes every hour. Set a timer to remind yourself.

Gardening: Gardening is a productive and enjoyable way to get some physical activity. Digging, weeding, and planting can be surprisingly good workouts.

Active Commuting: If you live relatively close to work or other destinations, consider walking or biking instead of driving. It's a great way to incorporate exercise into your daily routine.

Household Chores: Vacuuming, sweeping, mopping, and other household chores can be physically demanding. Consider these activities as part of your daily exercise.

Play with Pets: If you have pets, play with them. Activities like playing fetch with a dog or using a laser pointer with a cat can get you moving and provide entertainment for your furry friends.

Dance: Put on your favorite music and dance around while you cook, clean, or just for fun. Dancing is a fantastic way to get your heart rate up.

Active Meetings: If you have the flexibility, suggest walking meetings with colleagues. This can be a refreshing change from sitting in a conference room.

Park Farther Away: When you go to the store, park farther away from the entrance to get in some extra steps.

Take the Long Way: Whether you're at the mall, the office, or a large grocery store, intentionally take the longer route to your destination.

Use a Standing Desk: If possible, use a standing desk at work. Standing for part of the day can help reduce the negative effects of prolonged sitting.

Stretch Breaks: Incorporate stretching exercises into your daily routine. Stretching can help improve flexibility and reduce muscle tension.

Family Activities: Engage in physical activities with your family, such as bike rides, hikes, or playing sports together. It's a fun way to bond while staying active.

Consistency is key when it comes to incorporating physical activity into your daily life. Small, regular efforts add up over time and contribute to your overall health and well-being. Be creative and find opportunities to move throughout the day, even amid a busy schedule.

Chapter 6

Stress Management and Self-Care**

The Impact of Stress on Weight and Health

Stress can have a significant impact on both weight and overall health. The relationship between stress and these factors is complex and can vary from person to person, but there are several ways in which stress can affect weight and well-being:

Overeating and Weight Gain

- Emotional Eating: Many people turn to food for comfort when they're stressed, which can lead to emotional eating. Stress can trigger cravings for high-calorie, sugary, or fatty foods, often referred to as "comfort foods."

- Cortisol Release: Stress prompts the body to release cortisol, a hormone that can increase appetite, particularly for high-calorie foods. Cortisol also encourages the storage of fat, particularly in the abdominal area.

- Poor Food Choices: Stress can lead to poor dietary choices, such as reaching for convenient, processed foods that are typically high in calories, sugar, and unhealthy fats.

Weight Management Difficulties:
- Metabolism Changes: Chronic stress can affect your metabolism, making it more difficult to lose weight or maintain a healthy weight. This is partly due to cortisol's impact on metabolism.
- Sleep Disruption: Stress can disrupt sleep patterns, leading to inadequate or poor-quality sleep. Sleep deprivation is associated with weight gain and can affect hunger-regulating hormones, making you feel hungrier and less satisfied.

Impact on Health**:
- Chronic Diseases: Prolonged stress is associated with an increased risk of chronic diseases, including heart disease, diabetes, and obesity. These conditions can have a profound impact on overall health.
- Immune Function: Stress can weaken the immune system, making you more susceptible to illnesses and infections.

- Digestive Issues: Stress can affect the digestive system, leading to symptoms like indigestion, irritable bowel syndrome (IBS), and other gastrointestinal problems.

Behavior Changes:

- Physical Inactivity: Chronic stress may lead to decreased motivation for physical activity and exercise, contributing to a sedentary lifestyle.

- Alcohol and Substance Use: Some individuals may turn to alcohol, tobacco, or other substances as a way to cope with stress, which can have detrimental effects on health and weight.

Stress-Related Hormones:

- Insulin Resistance: Chronic stress can lead to insulin resistance, increasing the risk of type 2 diabetes.

- Leptin and Ghrelin: Stress can disrupt hormones that regulate appetite, leading to increased feelings of hunger and reduced feelings of fullness.

Managing stress effectively is crucial for both weight management and overall health. Here are some strategies to help mitigate the impact of stress:

- Regular Physical Activity: Exercise is an excellent way to combat stress and its effects on the body. It can help reduce cortisol levels, improve mood, and promote overall well-being.

- Mindfulness and Relaxation: Techniques like mindfulness meditation, deep breathing exercises, and yoga can help reduce stress and improve emotional well-being.

- Healthy Eating Habits: Focus on maintaining a balanced diet even during times of stress. Avoid overindulging in unhealthy comfort foods.

- Adequate Sleep: Prioritize good sleep hygiene to ensure you get enough restorative sleep.

- Social Support: Reach out to friends and family for support during stressful times. Talking to a therapist or counselor can also be beneficial.

- Time Management: Organize your tasks and responsibilities to reduce feelings of being overwhelmed.

- Hobbies and Leisure Activities: Engaging in enjoyable hobbies and activities can provide a healthy outlet for stress.

- Limiting Stimulants: Reduce or eliminate the consumption of stimulants like caffeine and nicotine, which can exacerbate stress.

It's important to recognize when stress is becoming chronic or overwhelming and seek professional help if needed. A healthcare provider or mental health professional can provide guidance and strategies for managing stress effectively to protect both your weight and your overall health.

Stress Reduction Techniques

Reducing stress is essential for promoting overall well-being and maintaining good health. There are numerous effective techniques and strategies you can incorporate into your daily routine to manage and reduce stress. Here are some stress reduction techniques to consider:

Deep Breathing: Practice deep breathing exercises to calm your nervous system. Inhale deeply through your nose for a count of four, hold for four, and then exhale through your mouth for four. Repeat several times.

Mindfulness Meditation: Engage in mindfulness meditation to stay present and reduce anxiety. Focus on your breath, bodily sensations, or a specific mantra. Even short daily sessions can be beneficial.

Progressive Muscle Relaxation: Tense and then relax each muscle group in your body, starting from your toes and working your way up to your head. This technique can help release physical tension associated with stress.

Yoga: Yoga combines physical postures, breath control, and meditation to promote relaxation and reduce stress. Regular practice can improve flexibility and reduce muscle tension.

Exercise: Engage in regular physical activity to release endorphins, the body's natural stress relievers. Activities like walking, jogging, swimming, or dancing can be effective.

Aromatherapy: Certain scents, such as lavender, chamomile, and eucalyptus, have calming properties. Use essential oils or scented candles to create a soothing atmosphere.

Journaling: Write down your thoughts and feelings in a journal. This can help you process emotions and gain clarity on stressors in your life.

Social Connection: Spend time with friends and loved ones. Sharing your thoughts and experiences with others can provide emotional support and reduce feelings of isolation.

Time Management: Organize your tasks and priorities to reduce feelings of being overwhelmed. Make to-do lists and break larger tasks into smaller, manageable steps.

Limit Screen Time: Set boundaries on the amount of time you spend on screens, including smartphones and computers. Excessive screen time can contribute to stress.

Nature and Outdoor Activities: Spend time in nature, whether it's a walk in the park, gardening, or hiking. Nature has a calming effect and can reduce stress levels.

Laughter: Watch a funny movie, read a humorous book, or spend time with people who make you laugh. Laughter can trigger the release of endorphins and reduce stress hormones.

Guided Imagery: Close your eyes and imagine a peaceful, calming place. Visualize the sights, sounds, and sensations. This technique can transport your mind away from stressors.

Limit Caffeine and Alcohol: Reduce your consumption of caffeine and alcohol, which can exacerbate stress and anxiety.

Seek Professional Help: If stress becomes overwhelming or persistent, consider talking to a mental health professional. Therapy, counseling, or stress management programs can provide valuable support.

Not all techniques work the same way for everyone, so it's essential to find what works best for you. Combining multiple strategies and incorporating them into your daily routine can help you effectively manage and reduce stress, leading to improved overall well-being.

The Importance of Quality Sleep

Quality sleep is vital for overall health and well-being. It plays a crucial role in various aspects of physical and mental health, and its importance cannot be overstated. Here are some key reasons why quality sleep is essential:

Physical Health:

Body Repair and Recovery: During deep sleep, the body undergoes essential repair and maintenance processes. Tissues and muscles are repaired, and the immune system is strengthened.

Hormone Regulation: Sleep helps regulate hormones that control appetite, metabolism, and stress. Lack of sleep can disrupt these hormone levels, leading to weight gain and increased stress.

Heart Health: Quality sleep is linked to a reduced risk of heart disease. It helps regulate blood pressure and lowers the risk of conditions like hypertension and stroke.

Immune Function: Adequate sleep is essential for a robust immune system. It enhances the body's ability to fight off infections and illnesses.

Blood Sugar Control: Sleep plays a role in blood sugar regulation. Poor sleep can lead to insulin resistance and an increased risk of type 2 diabetes.

Pain Management: Sleep is crucial for managing pain. It allows the body to release natural painkillers and reduces sensitivity to pain.

Mental Health:

Emotional Well-Being: Quality sleep is closely tied to emotional well-being. It helps regulate mood and reduces the risk of mood disorders like depression and anxiety.

Stress Reduction: A good night's sleep can lower stress levels and improve the ability to cope with daily challenges.

Cognitive Function: Sleep is essential for cognitive functions such as memory, attention, problem-solving, and creativity. It enhances learning and decision-making.

Mental Clarity: Adequate sleep improves mental clarity and focus, allowing for more productive and efficient daily activities.

Performance and Productivity:

Physical Performance: Athletes and individuals engaged in physical activities benefit from better physical performance and reduced risk of injury with quality sleep.

Work Productivity: Quality sleep enhances work productivity by improving concentration, problem-solving, and decision-making skills.

Creativity and Innovation: Restful sleep promotes creative thinking and innovation. It allows the brain to consolidate information and come up with new ideas.

Safety:

Reduced Accident Risk: Sleep-deprived individuals are more prone to accidents, both on the road and in the workplace. Quality sleep improves alertness and reduces the risk of accidents.

Longevity:

Increased Life Expectancy: Numerous studies have shown that those who consistently get quality sleep tend to live longer and have a higher quality of life in their later years.

To prioritize quality sleep, consider adopting healthy sleep habits, also known as sleep hygiene. This includes maintaining a consistent sleep schedule, creating a comfortable sleep environment, limiting exposure to screens before bedtime, and avoiding stimulants like caffeine and nicotine close to bedtime.

If you consistently experience sleep disturbances or have trouble achieving quality sleep, it's essential to consult with a healthcare provider or sleep specialist to address any underlying sleep disorders or conditions.

Incorporating quality sleep into your daily routine is an investment in your overall health and well-being. It supports physical health, mental clarity, emotional well-being, and overall vitality, helping you lead a happier and healthier life.

Chapter 7:

Strategies for Sustainable Weight Loss

Setting Up a Sustainable Routine

Creating a sustainable routine is key to maintaining a healthy and balanced lifestyle. Sustainability implies that your routine should be manageable, adaptable, and enjoyable in the long term. Here are steps to help you set up a sustainable routine:

Set Clear Goals: Begin by defining your goals. What do you want to achieve with your routine? Whether it's improving your health, managing stress, or increasing productivity, clear goals provide direction.

Start Small: Don't try to change everything at once. Start with one or two habits or activities that align with your goals. Once they become routine, add more as needed.

Create a Daily Schedule: Plan your day to include specific times for your routine activities. Consistency is key to making these activities a habit.

Prioritize Self-Care: Make self-care a non-negotiable part of your routine. This includes activities like exercise, meditation, quality sleep, and healthy eating.

Adaptability: Life is unpredictable, so build flexibility into your routine. Allow for changes and adjust your schedule when necessary. The goal is to maintain consistency over the long term, not perfection.

Time Management: Efficient time management helps you fit your routine into your day. Use tools like calendars, to-do lists, or productivity apps to help you stay organized.

Set Realistic Expectations: Ensure that your routine is realistic and achievable given your current circumstances. Setting overly ambitious goals can lead to frustration and burnout.

Monitor Progress: Track your progress toward your goals. This can help you stay motivated and adjust your routine as needed.

Accountability: Share your goals and routines with a friend, family member, or a support group. Having someone to hold you accountable can boost your commitment.

Incorporate Enjoyment: Choose activities and habits that you enjoy. This makes it more likely that you'll stick with your routine over the long term.

Reflect and Adjust: Regularly review your routine to see what's working and what needs improvement. Adjust as necessary to better align with your goals and current circumstances.

Self-Compassion: Be kind to yourself. If you miss a day or deviate from your routine occasionally, it's okay. Avoid self-criticism and focus on getting back on track.

Seek Professional Guidance: If your routine involves significant changes to your health or lifestyle, consider consulting with a healthcare professional or expert in the relevant field for guidance and support.

A sustainable routine supports your overall well-being and is adaptable to the various stages of life. It should enhance your quality of life rather than add stress. Building sustainable habits takes time and effort, so be patient with yourself and celebrate your achievements along the way.

Monitoring Progress and Adapting

Monitoring progress and adapting your routines and goals is essential to ensure you stay on track and continue to make positive changes in your life. Here are steps to effectively monitor progress and make necessary adaptations:

Set Clear Metrics: Define specific, measurable metrics related to your goals. This could include tracking the number of days you exercise, the amount of weight you've lost, or your daily meditation time.

Keep a Journal: Maintain a journal or diary to record your daily or weekly progress. Write down your achievements, setbacks, and how you feel about your routine.

Use Technology: There are numerous apps and digital tools available for tracking various aspects of your routine, such as fitness apps, calorie counters, and habit-tracking apps. These can provide valuable data and insights.

Regular Assessments: Schedule regular assessments to review your progress. This could be weekly, monthly, or quarterly, depending on your goals. Assessments allow you to see trends and make adjustments.

Celebrate Achievements: Celebrate your successes, no matter how small. Recognizing your achievements can boost motivation and reinforce positive habits.

Identify Challenges: Pay attention to any challenges or obstacles you encounter. Understanding what hinders your progress allows you to find solutions and make necessary adaptations.

Adjust Goals: If you find that your goals are too ambitious or not challenging enough, be willing to adjust them. Goals should be realistic and achievable, but they should also push you to grow.

Modify Routines: If certain aspects of your routine aren't working or feel monotonous, modify them. Change up your exercise routine, try new healthy recipes, or explore different relaxation techniques.

Seek Feedback: Reach out to a trusted friend, family member, or coach for feedback. They can provide a fresh perspective and suggest improvements.

Stay Informed: Continue learning about the areas relevant to your routine, whether it's nutrition, fitness, stress management, or any other aspect of your life. Staying informed can help you make more informed choices.

Listen to Your Body: Pay attention to your body's signals. If you're feeling fatigued, stressed, or unwell, it may be a sign that your routine needs adjustment. Rest and self-care are essential components of any successful routine.

Stay Flexible: Be flexible and willing to adapt as life circumstances change. What worked for you in one phase of life may not work in another. Flexibility allows you to maintain a sustainable routine.

Seek Professional Guidance: If you're working toward specific health or fitness goals, consider consulting with a healthcare provider, dietitian, personal trainer, or coach. They can offer expertise and guidance tailored to your needs.

Adaptation is a natural part of the journey toward your goals. It doesn't indicate failure but rather a willingness to learn and grow. By monitoring your progress and making thoughtful adaptations, you can create a routine that continues to serve your evolving needs and supports your long-term well-being.

Celebrating Milestones

Celebrating milestones is a crucial part of your personal growth and journey towards achieving your goals. Recognizing and celebrating your achievements, whether big or small, can provide motivation, boost self-esteem, and reinforce positive behaviors. Here's how to effectively celebrate your milestones:

Acknowledge Your Achievements: Take a moment to acknowledge what you've accomplished. Reflect on the effort, time, and dedication you put into reaching your milestone.

Set Specific Milestones: Break your larger goals into smaller, achievable milestones. Celebrating these smaller victories along the way can keep you motivated and focused on your long-term objectives. Reward Yourself: Consider rewarding yourself when you reach a milestone. This can be something meaningful to you, such as a treat, a small purchase, a day off, or a special activity you enjoy.

Share Your Success: Share your achievements with friends, family, or a supportive community. Celebrating with others can amplify the joy and provide a sense of accomplishment.

Capture the Moment: Take a photo, write in a journal, or create a scrapbook to commemorate the milestone. This allows you to preserve memories of your accomplishments.

Reflect on Your Journey: Use this time to reflect on the progress you've made, the lessons you've learned, and the personal growth you've experienced. Recognize how far you've come.

Set New Goals: After celebrating a milestone, consider setting new goals or revising existing ones. This keeps you motivated and maintains a sense of purpose.

Express Gratitude: Express gratitude for the support you've received along the way. Thank those who have helped and encouraged you.

Visualize Future Success: Use your milestone celebration as an opportunity to visualize your future success. This positive visualization can inspire you to continue striving for more.

Keep a Milestone Journal: Maintain a journal dedicated to your milestones and celebrations. Reviewing your achievements can be a powerful source of motivation.

Give Back: Consider giving back or paying it forward in some way. Celebrating by helping others or contributing to a cause you care about can be deeply fulfilling.

Stay Humble: While it's important to celebrate your accomplishments, remain humble and grounded.

Recognize that there is always room for growth and improvement.

Use Positive Self-Talk: Celebrate with positive self-talk. Remind yourself of your abilities, resilience, and determination that got you to this point.

Learn From Setbacks: If you encounter setbacks or challenges on your journey, view them as opportunities for growth and learning. Use them as stepping stones toward future milestones.

Celebrate Others' Achievements: Encourage and celebrate the achievements of those around you. Celebrating others can create a positive and supportive environment.

Celebrating milestones is not just about the result; it's also about appreciating the journey and recognizing your progress along the way. Each milestone you reach is a testament to your determination and commitment, and it deserves to be celebrated and cherished.

Chapter 8

Maintaining Your Achievements for Life

The Lifelong Commitment to Health

A lifelong commitment to health is a profound investment in your well-being and quality of life. It involves consistently making choices and adopting habits that promote physical, mental, and emotional health throughout all stages of life. Here are key principles for maintaining a lifelong commitment to health:

Prioritize Preventive Care: Regular check-ups, screenings, and vaccinations can detect potential health issues early and prevent them from escalating. Make these a routine part of your healthcare.

Maintain a Balanced Diet: Eat a variety of nutrient-rich foods, emphasizing fruits, vegetables, lean proteins, whole grains, and healthy fats. Avoid excessive consumption of processed foods, sugar, and unhealthy fats.

Stay Physically Active: Engage in regular physical activity, tailored to your age and fitness level. Incorporate aerobic, strength, flexibility, and balance exercises into your routine.

Quality Sleep: Prioritize getting sufficient and restful sleep each night. Create a comfortable sleep environment and establish consistent sleep patterns.

Manage Stress: Develop effective stress management techniques such as meditation, mindfulness, deep breathing, or yoga. Managing stress is crucial for mental and physical health.

Stay Hydrated: Drink an adequate amount of water daily to support bodily functions and overall well-being.

Limit Harmful Habits: Avoid smoking, excessive alcohol consumption, and drug use. These habits can have serious health consequences.

Cultivate Mental Well-Being: Foster mental health through activities that promote emotional resilience, such as therapy, journaling, or spending time in nature.

Social Connections: Maintain strong social connections and nurture meaningful relationships with friends and family. Social support is vital for emotional health.

Continual Learning: Cultivate a curious mind and engage in lifelong learning. Staying mentally active can help maintain cognitive function and prevent mental decline.

Regular Exercise: Incorporate regular physical activity into your life, even as you age. Adjust the intensity and type of exercise as needed to suit your abilities.

Mindful Eating: Practice mindful eating by savoring each bite and paying attention to hunger and fullness cues. Avoid emotional or mindless eating.

Stay Informed: Keep up to date with health-related information, research, and medical advancements. Being informed empowers you to make informed decisions about your health.

Preventative Measures: Follow recommended vaccinations, screenings, and preventative measures for age-related health conditions. Early detection and prevention are key.

Embrace Change: Be open to adapting your health practices and routines as you age. Recognize that your needs and abilities may change, and adjust accordingly.

Inspire Others: Share your commitment to health with others and inspire them to make positive changes in their lives. Supporting each other creates a healthier community.

Celebrate Achievements: Celebrate your health milestones and achievements, whether it's a successful fitness goal, improved eating habits, or better stress management.

A lifelong commitment to health is an ongoing journey that evolves with time and experience. It's about valuing your well-being, nurturing your body and mind, and making choices that enable you to lead a fulfilling and vibrant life throughout your lifetime.

Strategies for Preventing Weight Regain

Preventing weight regain can be challenging, but it's essential for long-term success in maintaining a healthier weight. After achieving your weight loss goals, here are some strategies to help you avoid regaining the weight:

Set Realistic Goals: Maintain realistic expectations about weight maintenance. Aim for a sustainable weight that aligns with your lifestyle and overall health.

Consistent Monitoring: Continue to monitor your weight regularly, ideally once a week. Early detection of weight changes allows you to address any gain promptly.

Nutrient-Dense Eating: Focus on nutrient-dense foods that provide essential vitamins, minerals, and fiber. Incorporate plenty of fruits, vegetables, lean proteins, whole grains, and healthy fats into your diet.

Mindful Eating: Practice mindful eating by paying attention to hunger and fullness cues. Avoid emotional or stress-related eating. Eat slowly and savor each bite.

Regular Physical Activity: Maintain a consistent exercise routine that includes a combination of aerobic, strength, and flexibility exercises. Aim for at least 150 minutes of moderate-intensity aerobic activity per week.

Stay Hydrated: Drink plenty of water throughout the day. Sometimes thirst can be mistaken for hunger.

Balanced Meals: Consume balanced meals with appropriate portion sizes. Avoid skipping meals, which can lead to overeating later in the day.

Plan Meals and Snacks: Plan your meals and snacks to avoid impulsive and unhealthy food choices. Prepare healthy snacks to have on hand when hunger strikes.

Limit Processed Foods: Minimize your intake of highly processed and sugary foods, which can contribute to weight gain and cravings.

Regular Sleep: Prioritize quality sleep as inadequate sleep can disrupt hunger-regulating hormones and increase the risk of weight gain.

Stress Management: Practice stress management techniques like meditation, yoga, deep breathing, or hobbies that help you relax and reduce stress-related eating.

Social Support: Continue seeking support from friends, family, or a support group. Having a support system can help you stay accountable.

Track Your Progress: Keep a journal of your eating habits, exercise routines, and any changes in your weight. This can help you identify patterns and make necessary adjustments.

Healthy Cooking: Learn to cook and prepare nutritious meals at home. Cooking your food gives you control over ingredients and portion sizes.

Recognize Triggers: Identify situations, emotions, or events that trigger unhealthy eating habits. Develop strategies to cope with these triggers without turning to food.

Be Patient and Forgiving: Understand that weight fluctuations are normal and may occur due to various factors, including water retention, hormones, and stress. Be patient with yourself and avoid self-criticism.

Regular Check-Ins: Schedule regular check-ins with a healthcare provider, dietitian, or fitness professional to assess your progress and adjust your plan as needed.

Maintenance Calories: Determine your maintenance calorie intake and adjust your eating habits to match it. Consuming excess calories, even from healthy foods, can lead to weight gain.

Celebrate Non-Scale Victories: Celebrate achievements that are not solely related to the number on the scale, such as improved fitness, increased energy levels, or better overall health.

Keep Learning: Stay informed about nutrition, exercise, and health-related topics. Continuously educate yourself to make informed choices.

Maintaining weight loss is an ongoing process that requires commitment and dedication. It's normal to face challenges along the way, but with a solid plan, a supportive environment, and a focus on long-term health, you can successfully prevent weight regain and enjoy the benefits of a healthier weight.

Adjusting Your Approach as You Age

As you age, it's essential to adjust your approach to health and well-being to accommodate the changes that naturally occur with time. Here are some key considerations and adjustments you can make to ensure a healthy and fulfilling life as you get older:

Physical Activity:

- Adjust Exercise Routine: Modify your exercise routine to match your age and physical condition. Focus on activities that support flexibility, balance, and strength, as these become more critical with age.

- Low-Impact Activities: Consider low-impact activities like swimming, cycling, or yoga to reduce the risk of injury to joints and bones.

- Regular Movement: Incorporate regular movement into your daily life, such as walking, gardening, or dancing. Staying active is essential for maintaining mobility.

Nutrition:

- Balanced Diet: Continue to prioritize a balanced diet rich in whole foods, but adjust your calorie intake to match your changing metabolism. Include more nutrient-dense foods to support overall health.

- Adequate Hydration: Pay attention to hydration as the sensation of thirst may diminish with age. Drink enough water to prevent dehydration.

- Dietary Supplements: Consult with a healthcare provider to determine if you need dietary supplements, such as vitamin D or calcium, which may become more important as you age.

Sleep**:

- Sleep Changes: Be aware that your sleep patterns may change with age. Focus on creating a comfortable sleep environment and maintaining consistent sleep routines.

Stress Management:

- Stress Reduction: Continue practicing stress reduction techniques like meditation, mindfulness, or relaxation exercises to support mental and emotional well-being.

Health Screenings:

- Regular Check-Ups: Maintain regular check-ups with healthcare providers for age-appropriate health screenings. These can help detect and manage age-related health conditions.

Social Connections**:

- Social Engagement: Stay socially engaged by maintaining and building relationships with friends and family. Social connections contribute to emotional well-being and overall happiness.

Mental Fitness**:

- Mental Stimulation: Engage in activities that stimulate your mind, such as reading, puzzles, or learning new skills. Cognitive health remains important throughout life.

Medication Management**:

- Medication Review: Regularly review your medications with a healthcare provider to ensure they are appropriate and safe for your age and health conditions.

Safety:

- Home Safety: Assess your living environment for safety hazards, especially if you live alone. Make necessary modifications to prevent accidents.

- Fall Prevention: Focus on fall prevention strategies, including exercise, balance training, and using assistive devices if needed.

Financial Planning:

- Retirement Planning: If you haven't already, consider retirement planning to ensure financial security in your later years.

Legal Documents:

- Estate Planning: Review and update your estate planning documents, such as wills, powers of attorney, and advance directives for healthcare.

Positive Mindset:

- Embrace Aging: Embrace the aging process with a positive mindset. Focus on the wisdom and experience that come with age, and continue to set and pursue meaningful goals.

Seek Professional Guidance**:

- Consult Experts: Seek advice from healthcare professionals, financial advisors, and legal experts when needed to ensure that your plans and decisions are in your best interest.

Adjusting your approach as you age is a proactive way to maintain your health, happiness, and overall quality of life. By staying informed, staying active, and staying connected, you can navigate the challenges and embrace the opportunities that come with each new stage of life.

Chapter 9

Inspirational Stories and Testimonials

Real-Life Success Stories

Real-life weight loss success stories are powerful examples of individuals who have made significant changes to improve their health and well-being through dedication, lifestyle changes, and determination. Here are a few real-life weight loss success stories:

Jared Fogle:- Jared Fogle became famous as the "Subway Guy" after losing an incredible 245 pounds by eating Subway sandwiches and making healthier choices. His transformation inspired many to consider healthier eating habits.

Chris Pratt:- Actor Chris Pratt went through a remarkable physical transformation for his roles in movies like "Guardians of the Galaxy." He lost weight and built muscle through rigorous exercise and a disciplined diet.

Ethan Suplee: Known for his roles in various films and TV shows, Ethan Suplee underwent a dramatic weight loss transformation. He lost over 200 pounds by adopting a healthier lifestyle and embracing physical fitness.

Mama June Shannon: Reality TV star Mama June Shannon documented her weight loss journey on the show "Mama June: From Not to Hot." She underwent surgery, adopted healthier eating habits, and engaged in exercise to lose a significant amount of weight.

John Goodman: Actor John Goodman lost a substantial amount of weight and adopted a healthier lifestyle after recognizing the importance of his health. He credited his weight loss to a change in diet and exercise.

Adele: The Grammy-winning singer Adele lost weight and underwent a physical transformation. While she didn't publicly disclose all the details of her journey, her dedication to healthier living inspired many fans.

These real-life weight loss success stories demonstrate that sustainable weight loss is possible with commitment, hard work, and a focus on overall health. Each individual's journey is unique, highlighting the importance of finding a weight loss approach that works for one's body and lifestyle. These stories serve as motivation for anyone striving to achieve their weight loss goals and improve their overall well-being.

Lessons Learned from Those Who Have Succeeded

Learning from those who have succeeded in weight loss can provide valuable insights and inspiration for your journey to a healthier weight. Here are some key lessons learned from individuals who have achieved lasting weight loss success:

Consistency is Key: Successful weight loss often comes from consistent, sustainable changes to eating habits and physical activity. Crash diets and extreme measures are less likely to lead to long-term success.

Set Realistic Goals: Setting achievable and realistic weight loss goals is essential. Small, incremental changes are more sustainable and less overwhelming.

Mindful Eating: Many successful individuals emphasize the importance of mindful eating. Paying attention to hunger and fullness cues, savoring each bite, and avoiding emotional eating can lead to healthier habits.

Find Enjoyable Exercise: Discover physical activities you genuinely enjoy. Whether it's dancing, hiking, swimming, or team sports, making exercise fun increases the likelihood of sticking with it.

Stay Accountable: Having a support system or an accountability partner can be highly effective. Sharing your goals with someone who can offer encouragement and motivation can make a significant difference.

Plan and Prep Meals: Planning and preparing meals in advance can help you make healthier food choices and avoid impulsive, less nutritious options.

Track Progress: Monitoring your progress through regular weigh-ins or keeping a food and exercise journal can help you stay on track and identify areas for improvement.

Embrace Variety: Incorporate a variety of foods into your diet to ensure you get a wide range of nutrients. Avoiding restrictive diets and enjoying diverse, balanced meals is more sustainable.

Learn from Setbacks: Weight loss journeys are rarely without setbacks. Instead of giving up when faced with challenges, learn from them and use setbacks as opportunities for growth.

Seek Professional Guidance: Consulting with a healthcare provider, registered dietitian, or personal trainer can provide personalized guidance tailored to your specific needs and goals.

Celebrate Non-Scale Victories: Focus on achievements beyond the number on the scale. Celebrate improved energy levels, better sleep, enhanced fitness, and increased self-confidence.

Perseverance Matters: Weight loss is a long-term commitment. Even if progress is slow, keep moving forward and stay patient. Success often comes to those who persist.

Avoid Comparison: Everyone's weight loss journey is unique. Avoid comparing your progress to others. Focus on your own goals and celebrate your successes.

Maintenance is Key: Weight maintenance is as important as weight loss. Developing strategies for maintaining your healthier weight is essential for long-term success.

Mindset Matters: Cultivate a positive and resilient mindset. Believe in your ability to achieve your goals and overcome challenges along the way.

Self-Care: Prioritize self-care in all aspects of your life. Managing stress, getting quality sleep, and nurturing your mental and emotional well-being are crucial for successful weight management.

Lifestyle, Not Diet: Shift your perspective from "dieting" to adopting a healthier lifestyle. Focus on making sustainable, lifelong changes rather than short-term fixes.

Share Your Journey: Sharing your journey with others, whether through social media or in-person support groups, can provide motivation and create a sense of accountability.

Know that each weight loss journey is personal, and what works for one person may not work for another. It's essential to find an approach that aligns with your preferences, needs, and values. Learning from those who have succeeded in weight loss can offer guidance and inspiration, but ultimately, your journey will be uniquely yours.

Finding Motivation in Others' Journeys

Finding motivation in others' weight loss journeys can be a powerful tool to inspire and sustain your efforts. Here are some ways to draw inspiration from the experiences of others:

Real-Life Success Stories: Read or watch real-life weight loss success stories. These stories often highlight the challenges people face, their strategies for overcoming them, and the positive impact of their transformation.

Social Media and Online Communities: Follow individuals or groups on social media platforms dedicated to health and fitness. You can connect with people who share their journeys, progress, tips, and support.

Join Support Groups: Participate in weight loss or fitness support groups, either in person or online. Sharing experiences and challenges with like-minded individuals can provide valuable motivation and encouragement.

Documented Transformations: Seek out documentaries or television shows that follow individuals on their weight loss journeys. These programs often showcase the emotional and physical transformations people undergo.

Health and Fitness Blogs: Explore blogs written by individuals who have successfully lost weight and maintained a healthier lifestyle. They often share practical advice and personal insights.

Before-and-After Photos: Before-and-after photos can be highly motivating. Seeing the visible changes in someone's appearance and hearing their story can boost your determination.

Quotes and Testimonials: Collect inspirational quotes and testimonials from people who have overcome weight-related challenges. Keep these reminders of success where you can see them daily.

Accountability Partners: Partner with a friend or family member who has similar health goals. You can motivate each other and celebrate milestones together.

Follow Influential Figures: Follow fitness trainers, nutritionists, or health experts who share their knowledge and the stories of their clients' successes.

Celebrities' Journeys: Learn about the weight loss journeys of celebrities who have openly discussed their transformations. Their visibility can serve as a reminder that anyone can achieve their goals.

Weekly Challenges: Consider participating in weekly or monthly challenges hosted by fitness influencers or groups. These challenges often provide structure and motivation to stay on track.

Visualize Your Success: Use others' success stories as a source of inspiration to visualize your success. Imagine how achieving your goals will positively impact your life.

Stay Connected: Keep up with the ongoing journeys of those you find motivating. Witnessing their continued success can help you maintain your motivation over time.

Share Your Progress: As you progress on your journey, consider sharing your own story and experiences with others. Your journey may inspire someone else just as you've been inspired.

Everyone's journey is unique, and it's essential to focus on your own goals and progress. While others' success can be motivating, avoid comparing yourself or setting unrealistic expectations. Use their stories as sources of encouragement and as evidence that positive change is achievable. Your determination and commitment will ultimately be the driving force behind your success.

Conclusion

In conclusion, "The Lasting Journey to a Healthier You: Sustainable Weight Loss Strategies after 40" serves as a comprehensive guide and a source of inspiration for anyone embarking on the path to improved health and well-being, particularly for those navigating the challenges of weight management beyond the age of 40.

Throughout this book, we have explored the significance of age 40 as a pivotal moment when our bodies undergo transformations that demand a thoughtful approach to health. We've delved into the importance of setting realistic goals, nurturing the right mindset, and understanding the physiological changes, such as shifts in metabolism and hormonal fluctuations, that impact our bodies as we age.

From the critical role of muscle mass in weight management to addressing emotional eating and cultivating mindful eating habits, we've uncovered valuable strategies to help you not only shed unwanted pounds but also develop a lasting relationship with your health. Moreover, we've discussed the significance of incorporating age-appropriate exercise routines and the importance of strength training and cardiovascular health in maintaining vitality.

This book has also explored the impact of stress on both weight and overall well-being, providing strategies to manage and reduce stress effectively. We've highlighted the crucial role of quality sleep in your health journey and shared insights on setting up a sustainable routine that aligns with your goals and lifestyle.

Monitoring progress, adapting as needed, and celebrating milestones have been emphasized as essential practices for long-term success. By drawing inspiration from real-life success stories and those who have achieved lasting transformations, you are reminded that your journey is unique and entirely achievable.

In the quest for a healthier you after 40, remember that success is not solely defined by a number on the scale but by the enduring changes you make to nurture your well-being. The commitment you make to your health is a lifelong endeavor—one that requires patience, perseverance, and a deep understanding of your body and mind.

As you embark on your lasting journey to a healthier you, know that this book is a roadmap, a trusted companion, and a source of motivation. We hope that the sustainable weight loss strategies, lifestyle adjustments, and mindset shifts presented here empower you to create positive, lasting change in your life.

May your journey be filled with renewed energy, vibrant health, and a profound sense of well-being. Here's to the lasting transformation you are about to embark upon—the journey to a healthier, happier, and more fulfilled you, not just today, but for the years to come.

Appendix: Resources and Additional Reading

In the appendix of "The Lasting Journey to a Healthier You: Sustainable Weight Loss Strategies after 40," you'll find a curated list of valuable resources and additional reading materials to support your ongoing journey to better health and sustainable weight management. These resources are designed to complement the knowledge and strategies discussed in the main content of the book, providing you with further insights, guidance, and support.

Please note that this list is not exhaustive, and there are many more resources available to explore based on your specific interests and needs. Consider this a starting point for your continued exploration and education on topics related to health, fitness, nutrition, and well-being.

Books:

- "The Obesity Code: Unlocking the Secrets of Weight Loss" by Dr. Jason Fung

- "Mindless Eating: Why We Eat More Than We Think" by Brian Wansink, Ph.D.
- "Younger Next Year: Live Strong, Fit, and Sexy - Until You're 80 and Beyond" by Chris Crowley and Henry S. Lodge, M.D.
- "The Blue Zones: Lessons for Living Longer From the People Who've Lived the Longest" by Dan Buettner
- "The Power of Habit: Why We Do What We Do in Life and Business" by Charles Duhigg

Websites and Online Resources:

- National Institute on Aging (NIA) - Provides valuable information on aging-related topics, health, and nutrition.
- Centers for Disease Control and Prevention (CDC) - Offers resources on healthy living, nutrition, and physical activity.
- Academy of Nutrition and Dietetics - Features nutrition tips and resources for maintaining a healthy diet.
- American Council on Exercise (ACE) - Offers exercise tips, workout routines, and fitness resources.

Apps and Tools:
- MyFitnessPal - A popular app for tracking nutrition and exercise, helping you stay on top of your health goals.
- Fitbit - A wearable fitness tracker that monitors activity, sleep, and more.
- Calm - A meditation and mindfulness app for stress reduction and relaxation.
- Headspace - Another mindfulness and meditation app with guided sessions for improved mental well-being.
- Sleep Cycle - An app that tracks your sleep patterns and offers insights for better sleep quality.

Support Groups and Communities:**
- Join local or online support groups focused on weight loss, health, and fitness.
- Consider seeking out social media groups or forums where individuals share their experiences and provide encouragement.

Professional Guidance:**
- Consult with a registered dietitian or nutritionist for personalized dietary advice.
- Seek the guidance of a personal trainer or fitness coach to develop a tailored exercise plan.

- Connect with a healthcare provider for medical assessments and advice on managing health conditions.

Educational Courses:

- Explore online courses or workshops related to nutrition, fitness, stress management, and healthy aging.